Best Air

Cookbook

Quick and Easy Recipes for Beginners.
Improve your Lifestyle with Affordable
and Healthy Dishes.
Fry, Grill, Roast, and Bake Everyday.

Amanda Grace

TABLE OF CONTENTS

INTRODUCTION

The Air Fryer comes with 12-preset cooking functions. While using these functions you never need to worry about the time and temperature settings all preset or you can recall your last used settings using these functions.

Air Fry

Air Fry: This is one of the healthy cooking functions used to air fry your favorite foods like snacks with very little oil. Using this function, you can make your food crispy from the outside and tender, juicy from the inside.

First set the crispier tray at the 4th rack position.

The heat comes from side heating elements.

While using this function air fryer fan is always on.

Toast

Toast: Using this function you can easily toast your white or brown bread. It makes your bread brown and nice crisp on both sides.

First set the pizza rack at the 2nd rack position.

Select the desire darkness level between 1-5.

Select the desired number of bread slices between 1-6.

Bagel

Bagel: This function works the same as the toast function. You need to set your bagel slice over the pizza rack. It makes your bagel nice crisp and brown on both sides.

First set the pizza rack at the 2nd rack position.

Select the desire darkness level between 1-5.

Select the desired number of bagel slices between 1-6.

Pizza

Pizza: Using this function you can make a perfect homemade pizza or you can also make frozen pizza.

First set the pizza rack at the 5th rack position.

While using this function air fryer fan is always on.

Bake

Bake: This function is ideal for baking your favorite cake, cookies, pastries, pies, and more.

First set your baking tray or pizza rack at the 5th rack position.

While using this function air fryer fan can turn off.

Broil

Broil: Using this function you can broil your favorite sandwiches or melt cheese over burgers.

First set your baking pan or pizza rack on 1st or 2nd rack position.

While using this function air fryer fan can turn off.

Rotisserie

Rotisserie: It is also known as the split roasting method to roast your whole chicken using rotisserie tools. It makes your chicken crisp from the outside and tender, juicy from the inside.

Use rotisserie split accessories and set it at the 3rd rotisserie slot position.

While using this function air fryer fan can turn off.

Slow Cook

Slow Cook: This function cooks your food for a longer time especially great for tough meat cuts. It makes your tough meats tender and juicy.

First set the pizza rack at 6th position.

While using this function air fryer fan is always on.

Roast

Roast: This function is ideal for roasting a large piece of poultry or meat and it gives even cooking results.

First set pizza rack at 5th rack position.

While using this function air fryer fan is always on.

Dehydrate

Dehydrate: Using this function you can dehydrate your favorite meat, vegetable, and fruit slices.

First set the crisper tray at 1st, 4th, and 5th position.

While using this function air fryer fan is always on.

Reheat

Reheat: Using this function you can reheat your food without searing.

First set pizza rack at 5th rack position.

While using this function air fryer fan is always on.

Warm

Warm: This setting is ideal to keep your food warm by maintaining a safe temperature (160°F) until it is ready to serve.

First set baking pan, pizza rack, or crisper tray at 5th rack position.

While using this function air fryer fan can turn off.

BREAKFAST

Cheesy Bell Pepper Eggs

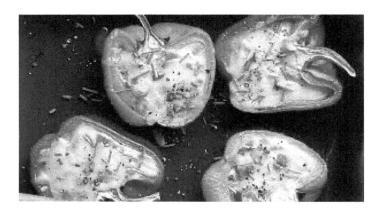

Preparation Time: 10 minutes

Cooking Time: 15 minutes

Servings: 4

Ingredients:

- 4 medium green bell peppers
- 3 ounces cooked ham, chopped
- ¼ medium onion, peeled and chopped
- 8 large eggs
- 1 cup mild Cheddar cheese

Directions:

1. Cut the tops off each bell pepper. Remove the seeds and the white membranes with a small knife. Place ham and onion into each pepper.

2. Crack 2 eggs into each pepper. Top with ¼ cup cheese per pepper. Place into the air fryer basket.

3. Adjust the temperature to 390°F and set the timer for 15 minutes.

4. When fully cooked, peppers will be tender and eggs will be firm. Serve immediately.

Nutrition: Calories: 314 Protein: 24.9 g Fiber: 1.7 g Net carbohydrates: 4.6 g Fat: 18.6 g Sodium: 621 mg Carbohydrates: 6.3 g Sugar: 3.0 g

Spaghetti Squash Fritters

Preparation Time: 15 minutes

Cooking Time: 8 minutes

Servings: 4

Ingredients:

- 2 cups cooked spaghetti squash
- 2 tablespoons unsalted butter, softened
- 1 large egg
- ¼ cup blanched finely ground almond flour
- 2 stalks green onion, sliced
- ½ teaspoon garlic powder
- 1 teaspoon dried parsley

Directions:

1. Remove excess moisture from the squash using a cheesecloth or kitchen towel.
2. Mix all ingredients in a large bowl. Form into four patties.
3. Cut a piece of parchment to fit your air fryer basket. Place each patty on the parchment and place into the air fryer basket.

4. Adjust the temperature to 400°F and set the timer for 8 minutes.

5. Flip the patties halfway through the cooking time. Serve warm.

Nutrition: Calories: 131 Protein: 3.8 g Fiber: 2.0 g Net carbohydrates: 5.1 g Fat: 10.1 g Sodium: 33 mg Carbohydrates: 7.1 g Sugar: 2.3 g

Cauliflower Roast Crunch

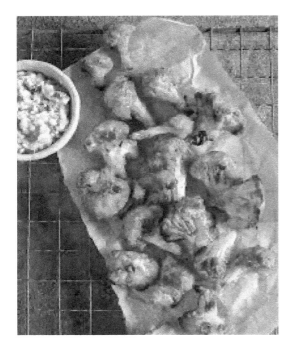

Preparation Time 10 Minutes

Cooking Time 10 Minutes

Servings: 4

Ingredients

- 1 medium cauliflower head, leaves removed
- ¼ cup olive oil
- 1 teaspoon red pepper, crushed
- ½ cup water
- 2 tablespoons capers, rinsed and minced
- ½ cup parmesan cheese, grated

- 1 tablespoon fresh parsley, chopped

Directions

1. Prepare the Air fryer by adding water and place the cook and crisp basket inside the pot
2. Cut an "X" on the head of cauliflower by using a knife and slice it about halfway down
3. Take a basket and transfer the cauliflower in it
4. Then put on the pressure lid and seal it and set it on low pressure for 3 minutes
5. Add olive oil, capers, garlic, and crushed red pepper into it and mix them well
6. Once the cauliflower is cooked, do a quick release and remove the lid
7. Pour in the oil and spice mixture on the cauliflower
8. Spread equally on the surface then sprinkle some Parmesan cheese from the top
9. Close the pot with crisping lid. Set it on Air Crisp mode to 390 degrees F for 10 minutes
10. Once done, remove the cauliflower flower the Air fryer transfer it into a serving plate

11.   Cut it up into pieces and transfer them to serving plates

12.   Sprinkle fresh parsley from the top. Serve and enjoy!

Nutrition: Calories: 119 Fat: 10g Carbohydrates: 5g Protein: 2.2g

Spinach Quiche

Preparation Time 10 Minutes

Cooking Time 33 Minutes

Servings: 4

Ingredients

- 1 tablespoon butter, melted
- 1 pack frozen spinach, thawed
- 5 organic eggs, beaten
- Salt and pepper to taste
- 3 cups Monterey Jack Cheese, shredded

Directions

1. Set your Air fryer to Sauté mode and let it heat up, add butter and let the butter melt
2. Add spinach and Sauté for 3 minutes, transfer the Sautéed spinach to a bowl
3. Add eggs, cheese, salt and pepper to a bowl and mix it well
4. Transfer the mixture to greased quiche molds and transfer the mold to your Foodi
5. Close lid and choose the "Bake/Roast" mode and let it cook for 30 minutes at 360 degrees F

6. Once done, open lid and transfer the dish out. Cut into wedges and serve. Enjoy!

Nutrition: Calories: 349 Fat: 27g Carbohydrates: 3.2g Protein: 23g

Broccoli Casserole

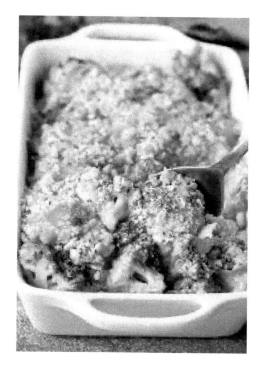

Preparation Time 10 Minutes

Cooking Time 7 Minutes

Servings: 4

Ingredients

- 1 tablespoon extra-virgin olive oil
- 1-pound broccoli, cut into florets
- 1-pound cauliflower, cut into florets
- ¼ cup almond flour
- 2 cups coconut milk

- ½ teaspoon ground nutmeg
- Pinch of pepper
- 1 and ½ cup shredded Gouda cheese, divided

Directions

1. Pre-heat your Air fryer by setting it to Sauté mode
2. Add olive oil and let it heat up, add broccoli and cauliflower
3. Take a medium bowl stir in almond flour, coconut milk, nutmeg, pepper, 1 cup cheese and add the mixture to your Air fryer
4. Top with ½ cup cheese and lock lid, cook on high pressure for 5 minutes
5. Release pressure naturally over 10 minutes. Serve and enjoy!

Nutrition: Calories: 373 Fat: 32g Carbohydrates: 6g Protein: 16g

Asparagus Soup

Preparation Time 10 Minutes

Cooking Time 10 Minutes

Servings: 4

Ingredients

- 1 tablespoon olive oil
- 3 green onions, sliced crosswise into ¼ inch pieces
- 1-pound asparagus, tough ends removed, cut into 1-inch pieces
- 4 cups vegetable stock
- 1 tablespoon unsalted butter
- 1 tablespoon almond flour
- 2 teaspoon salt
- 1 teaspoon white pepper
- ½ cup heavy cream

Directions

1. Set your Air fryer to "Sauté" mode and add oil, let it heat up
2. Add green onions and Sauté for a few minutes, add asparagus and stock

3. Lock lid and cook on high pressure for 5 minutes

4. Take a small saucepan and place it over low heat, add butter, flour and stir until the mixture foams and turns into a golden beige, this is your blond roux

5. Remove from heat. Release pressure naturally over 10 minutes

6. Open lid and add roux, salt and pepper to the soup

7. Use an immersion blender to puree the soup

8. Taste and season accordingly, swirl in cream and enjoy!

Nutrition: Calories: 192 Fat: 14g Carbohydrates: 8g Protein: 6g

Pumpkin Puree

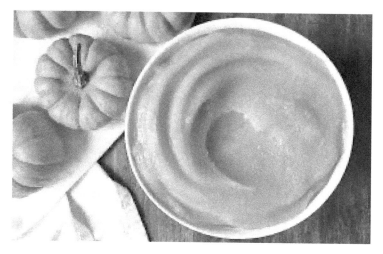

Preparation Time 10 Minutes

Cooking Time 15 Minutes

Servings: 2

Ingredients

- 2 pounds small sized pumpkin, halved and seeded
- ½ cup water
- Salt and pepper to taste

Directions

1. Add water to your Air fryer, place steamer rack in the pot

2. Add pumpkin halves to the rack and lock lid, cook on high pressure for 13-15 minutes
3. Once done, quick release pressure and let the pumpkin cool
4. Once done, scoop out flesh into a bowl
5. Blend using an immersion blender and season with salt and pepper. Serve and enjoy!

Nutrition: Calories: 112 Fat: 2g Carbohydrates: 7g Protein: 2g

Veggie and Bacon Delight

Preparation Time 5 Minutes

Cooking Time 25 Minutes

Servings: 4

Ingredients

- 1 green bell pepper, chopped
- 4 bacon slices
- ½ cup parmesan cheese
- 1 tablespoon avocado mayonnaise
- 2 scallions, chopped

Directions

1. Arrange your bacon slices in your Air fryer pot and top them up with avocado mayo, scallions, bell peppers, parmesan cheese
2. Close lid and select the Bake/Roast mode, set timer to 25 minutes and temperature to 365 degrees F. Let it bake and remove the dish after 25 minutes. Serve and enjoy!

Nutrition: Calories: 197 Fat: 13g Carbohydrates: 5g Protein: 14g

Scrambled Cheese and Broccoli

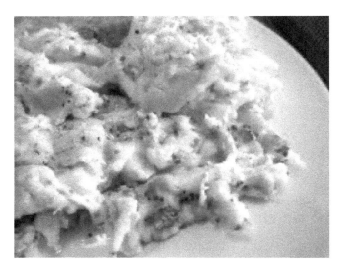

Preparation Time 10 Minutes

Cooking Time 5 Minutes

Servings: 4

Ingredients

- 1 pack, 12 ounces frozen broccoli florets
- 2 tablespoons butter
- salt and pepper
- 8 whole eggs
- 2 tablespoons milk
- ¾ cup white cheddar cheese, shredded
- Crushed red pepper

Directions

1. Add butter and broccoli to your Air fryer

2. Season with salt and pepper according to your taste

3. Set the Ninja to Medium Pressure mode and let it cook for about 10 minutes, covered, making sure to keep stirring the broccoli from time to time

4. Take a medium sized bowl and add crack in the eggs, beat the eggs gently

5. Pour milk into the eggs and give it a nice stir

6. Add the egg mixture into the Ninja over broccoli and gently stir, cook for 2 minutes, uncovered

7. Once the egg has settled in, add cheese and sprinkle red pepper, black pepper, and salt

8. Enjoy with bacon strips if you prefer!

Nutrition: Calories: 184 Fat: 12g Carbohydrates: 5g Protein: 12g

Scrambled Tofu and Onion

Preparation Time 8 Minutes

Cooking Time 12 Minutes

Servings: 4

Ingredients

- 4 tablespoons butter
- 2 tofu blocks, pressed and cubed in to 1-inch pieces
- Salt and pepper to taste
- 1 cup cheddar cheese, grated
- 2 medium onions, sliced

Directions

1. Take a bowl and add tofu, season with salt and pepper
2. Set your Foodi to Sauté mode and add butter, let it melt
3. Add onions and Sauté for 3 minutes. Add seasoned tofu and cook for 2 minutes more
4. Add cheddar and gently stir
5. Lock the lid and bring down the Air Crisp mode, let the dish cook on "Air Crisp" mode for 3

minutes at 340 degrees F. Once done, take the dish out, serve and enjoy!

Nutrition: Calories: 184 Fat: 12g Carbohydrates: 5g Protein: 12g

LUNCH

Mozzarella Walnut Stuffed Mushrooms

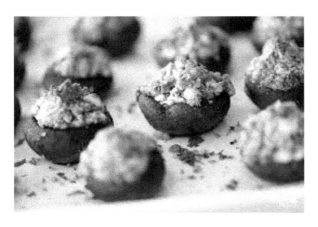

Preparation time: 5 minutes

Cooking time: 10 minutes

Servings: 4

Ingredients

- 4 large portobello mushrooms

- 1 tablespoon canola oil

- ½ cup shredded Mozzarella cheese

- ¹/₃ cup minced walnuts
- 2 tablespoons chopped fresh parsley
- Cooking spray

Directions

1. Spritz the perforated pan with cooking spray.
2. On a clean work surface, remove the mushroom stems. Scoop out the gills with a spoon and discard. Coat the mushrooms with canola oil. Top each mushroom evenly with the shredded Mozzarella cheese, followed by the minced walnuts.
3. Arrange the mushrooms in the perforated pan.
4. Select Roast. Set temperature to 350ºF (180ºC) and set time to 10 minutes. Press Start to begin preheating.
5. Once preheated, place the pan into the oven.
6. When cooking is complete, the mushroom should be golden brown.
7. Transfer the mushrooms to a plate and sprinkle the parsley on top for garnish before serving.

Nutrition: Calories 79 Carbs 7 g Protein 5 g Fat 3 g

Tomato-Stuffed Portobello Mushrooms

Preparation time: 5 minutes

Cooking time: 8 minutes

Servings: 4

Ingredients

- 4 portobello mushrooms, stem removed
- 1 tablespoon olive oil
- 1 tomato, diced
- ½ green bell pepper, diced
- ½ small red onion, diced
- ½ teaspoon garlic powder
- Salt and black pepper, to taste
- ½ cup grated Mozzarella cheese

Directions

1. Using a spoon to scoop out the gills of the mushrooms and discard them. Brush the mushrooms with the olive oil.

2. In a mixing bowl, stir together the remaining ingredients except the Mozzarella cheese. Using

a spoon to stuff each mushroom with the filling and scatter the Mozzarella cheese on top.

3. Arrange the mushrooms in the perforated pan.
4. Select Roast. Set temperature to 330ºF (166ºC) and set time to 8 minutes. Press Start to begin preheating.
5. Once preheated, place the pan into the oven.
6. When cooking is complete, the cheese should be melted.
7. Serve warm.

Nutrition: Calories 79 Carbs 7 g Protein 5 g Fat 3 g

Spinach-Stuffed Beefsteak Tomatoes

Preparation time: 10 minutes

Cooking time: 18 minutes

Servings: 4

Ingredients

- 4 medium beefsteak tomatoes, rinsed
- ½ cup grated carrot
- 1 medium onion, chopped
- 1 garlic clove, minced
- 2 teaspoons olive oil
- 2 cups fresh baby spinach
- ¼ cup crumbled low-sodium feta cheese
- ½ teaspoon dried basil

Directions

1. On your cutting board, cut a thin slice off the top of each tomato. Scoop out a ¼- to ½-inch-thick tomato pulp and place the tomatoes upside down on paper towels to drain. Set aside.

2. Stir together the carrot, onion, garlic, and olive oil in a baking pan.

3. Select Bake. Set temperature to 350ºF (180ºC) and set time to 5 minutes. Press Start to begin preheating.

4. Once preheated, place the pan into the oven. Stir the vegetables halfway through.

5. When cooking is complete, the carrot should be crisp-tender.

6. Remove the pan from the oven and stir in the spinach, feta cheese, and basil.

7. Spoon ¼ of the vegetable mixture into each tomato and transfer the stuffed tomatoes to the oven. Set time to 13 minutes on Bake.

8. When cooking is complete, the filling should be hot and the tomatoes should be lightly caramelized.

9. Let the tomatoes cool for 5 minutes and serve.

Nutrition: Calories 79 Carbs 7 g Protein 5 g Fat 3 g

Breaded Zucchini Chips with Parmesan

Preparation time: 5 minutes

Cooking time: 14 minutes

Servings: 4

Ingredients

- 2 egg whites
- Salt and black pepper, to taste
- ½ cup seasoned bread crumbs
- 2 tablespoons grated Parmesan cheese
- ¼ teaspoon garlic powder
- 2 medium zucchinis, sliced
- Cooking spray

Directions

1. Spritz the perforated pan with cooking spray.

2. In a bowl, beat the egg whites with salt and pepper. In a separate bowl, thoroughly combine the bread crumbs, Parmesan cheese, and garlic powder.

3. Dredge the zucchini slices in the egg white, then coat in the bread crumb mixture.

4. Arrange the zucchini slices in the perforated pan.

5. Select Air Fry. Set temperature to 400ºF (205ºC) and set time to 14 minutes. Press Start to begin preheating.

6. Once preheated, place the pan into the oven. Flip the zucchini halfway through.

7. When cooking is complete, the zucchini should be tender.

8. Remove from the oven to a plate and serve.

Nutrition: Calories 79 Carbs 7 g Protein 5 g Fat 3 g

Rice and Olives Stuffed Peppers

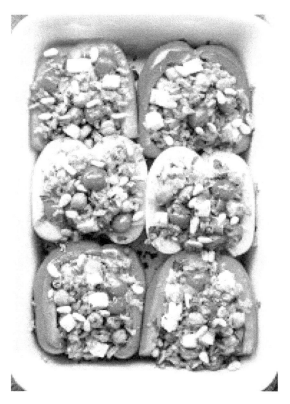

Preparation time: 5 minutes

Cooking time: 16 to 17 minutes

Servings: 4

Ingredients

- 4 red bell peppers, tops sliced off

- 2 cups cooked rice

- 1 cup crumbled feta cheese

- 1 onion, chopped

- ¼ cup sliced kalamata olives
- ¾ cup tomato sauce
- 1 tablespoon Greek seasoning
- Salt and black pepper, to taste
- 2 tablespoons chopped fresh dill, for serving

Directions

1. Microwave the red bell peppers for 1 to 2 minutes until tender.

2. When ready, transfer the red bell peppers to a plate to cool.

3. Mix the cooked rice, feta cheese, onion, kalamata olives, tomato sauce, Greek seasoning, salt, and pepper in a medium bowl and stir until well combined.

4. Divide the rice mixture among the red bell peppers and transfer to a greased baking dish.

5. Select Bake. Set temperature to 360ºF (182ºC) and set time to 15 minutes. Press Start to begin preheating.

6. Once preheated, place the baking dish into the oven.

7. When cooking is complete, the rice should be heated through and the vegetables should be soft.

8. Remove from the oven and serve with the dill sprinkled on top.

Nutrition: Calories 79 Carbs 7 g Protein 5 g Fat 3 g

Potato and Asparagus Platter

Preparation time: 5 minutes

Cooking time: 26 minutes

Servings: 5

Ingredients

- 4 medium potatoes, cut into wedges
- Cooking spray
- 1 bunch asparagus, trimmed
- 2 tablespoons olive oil
- Salt and pepper, to taste
- Cheese Sauce:
- ¼ cup crumbled cottage cheese
- ¼ cup buttermilk
- 1 tablespoon whole grain mustard
- Salt and black pepper, to taste

Directions

1. Spritz the perforated pan with cooking spray.
2. Put the potatoes in the perforated pan.
3. Select Roast. Set temperature to 400ºF (205ºC) and set time to 20 minutes. Press Start to begin preheating.

4. Once preheated, place the pan into the oven. Stir the potatoes halfway through.

5. When cooking is complete, the potatoes should be golden brown.

6. Remove the potatoes from the oven to a platter. Cover the potatoes with foil to keep warm. Set aside.

7. Place the asparagus in the perforated pan and drizzle with the olive oil. Sprinkle with salt and pepper.

8. Select Roast. Set temperature to 400ºF (205ºC) and set time to 6 minutes. Place the pan into the oven. Stir the asparagus halfway through.

9. When cooking is complete, the asparagus should be crispy.

10.   Meanwhile, make the cheese sauce by stirring together the cottage cheese, buttermilk, and mustard in a small bowl. Season as needed with salt and pepper.

11.   Transfer the asparagus to the platter of potatoes and drizzle with the cheese sauce. Serve immediately.

Nutrition: Calories 79 Carbs 7 g Protein 5 g Fat 3 g

Pepper-Stuffed Portobellos

Preparation time: 15 minutes

Cooking time: 15 minutes

Servings: 4

Ingredients

- 4 tablespoons sherry vinegar or white wine vinegar
- 6 garlic cloves, minced, divided
- 1 tablespoon fresh thyme leaves
- 1 teaspoon Dijon mustard
- 1 teaspoon kosher salt, divided
- ¼ cup plus 3¼ teaspoons extra-virgin olive oil, divided
- 8 portobello mushroom caps, each about 3 inches across, patted dry
- 1 small red or yellow bell pepper, thinly sliced
- 1 small green bell pepper, thinly sliced
- 1 small onion, thinly sliced
- ¼ teaspoon red pepper flakes
- Freshly ground black pepper, to taste
- 4 ounces (113 g) shredded Fontina cheese

Directions

1. Stir together the vinegar, 4 minced garlic cloves, thyme, mustard, and ½ teaspoon of kosher salt in a small bowl. Slowly pour in ¼ cup of olive oil, whisking constantly, or until an emulsion is formed. Reserve 2 tablespoons of the marinade and set aside.

2. Put the mushrooms in a resealable plastic bag and pour in the marinade. Seal and shake the bag, coating the mushrooms in the marinade. Transfer the mushrooms to the sheet pan, gill-side down.

3. Put the remaining 2 minced garlic cloves, bell peppers, onion, red pepper flakes, remaining ½ teaspoon of salt, and black pepper in a medium bowl. Drizzle with the remaining 3¼ teaspoons of olive oil and toss well. Transfer the bell pepper mixture to the sheet pan.

4. Select Roast. Set temperature to 375ºF (190ºC) and set time to 12 minutes. Press Start to begin preheating.

5. Once preheated, place the pan into the oven.

6. After 7 minutes, remove the pan and stir the peppers and flip the mushrooms. Return the pan to the oven and continue cooking for 5 minutes.

7. Remove the pan from the oven and place the pepper mixture onto a cutting board and coarsely chop.

8. Brush both sides of the mushrooms with the reserved 2 tablespoons marinade. Stuff the caps evenly with the pepper mixture. Scatter the cheese on top.

9. Select Broil. Set temperature to 400ºF (205ºC) and set time to 3 minutes. Place the pan into the oven.

10. When done, the mushrooms should be tender and the cheese should be melted.

11. Serve warm.

Nutrition: Calories 79 Carbs 7 g Protein 5 g Fat 3 g

Chickpea-Stuffed Bell Peppers

Preparation time: 10 minutes

Cooking time: 18 minutes

Servings: 4

Ingredients

- 4 medium red, green, or yellow bell peppers, halved and deseeded
- 4 tablespoons extra-virgin olive oil, divided
- ½ teaspoon kosher salt, divided
- 1 (15-ounce / 425-g) can chickpeas
- 1½ cups cooked white rice
- ½ cup diced roasted red peppers
- ¼ cup chopped parsley
- ½ small onion, finely chopped
- 3 garlic cloves, minced
- ½ teaspoon cumin
- ¼ teaspoon freshly ground black pepper
- ¾ cup panko bread crumbs

Directions

1. Brush the peppers inside and out with 1 tablespoon of olive oil. Season the insides with

¼ teaspoon of kosher salt. Arrange the peppers on the sheet pan, cut side up.

2. Place the chickpeas with their liquid into a large bowl. Lightly mash the beans with a potato masher. Sprinkle with the remaining ¼ teaspoon of kosher salt and 1 tablespoon of olive oil. Add the rice, red peppers, parsley, onion, garlic, cumin, and black pepper to the bowl and stir to incorporate.

3. Divide the mixture among the bell pepper halves.

4. Stir together the remaining 2 tablespoons of olive oil and panko in a small bowl. Top the pepper halves with the panko mixture.

5. Select Roast. Set temperature to 375ºF (190ºC) and set time to 18 minutes. Press Start to begin preheating.

6. Once preheated, place the pan into the oven.

7. When done, the peppers should be slightly wrinkled, and the panko should be golden brown.

8. Remove from the oven and serve on a plate.

Nutrition: Calories 79 Carbs 7 g Protein 5 g Fat 3 g

Stuffed Bell Peppers with Cream Cheese

Preparation time: 5 minutes

Cooking time: 15 minutes

Servings: 2

Ingredients

- 2 bell peppers, tops and seeds removed
- Salt and pepper, to taste
- $^2/_3$ cup cream cheese
- 2 tablespoons mayonnaise
- 1 tablespoon chopped fresh celery stalks
- Cooking spray

Directions

1. Spritz the perforated pan with cooking spray.
2. Place the peppers in the perforated pan.
3. Select Roast. Set temperature to 400ºF (205ºC) and set time to 10 minutes. Press Start to begin preheating.
4. Once preheated, place the pan into the oven. Flip the peppers halfway through.

5. When cooking is complete, the peppers should be crisp-tender.
6. Remove from the oven to a plate and season with salt and pepper.
7. Mix the cream cheese, mayo, and celery in a small bowl and stir to incorporate. Evenly stuff the roasted peppers with the cream cheese mixture with a spoon. Serve immediately.

Nutrition: Calories 79 Carbs 7 g Protein 5 g Fat 3 g

Mozzarella Tomato-Stuffed Squash

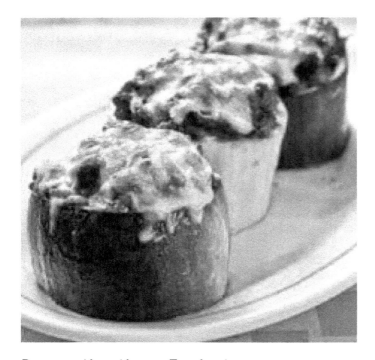

Preparation time: 5 minutes

Cooking time: 30 minutes

Servings: 4

Ingredients

- 1 pound (454 g) butternut squash, ends trimmed
- 2 teaspoons olive oil, divided
- 6 grape tomatoes, halved
- 1 poblano pepper, cut into strips

- Salt and black pepper, to taste
- ¼ cup grated Mozzarella cheese

Directions

1. Using a large knife, cut the squash in half lengthwise on a flat work surface. This recipe just needs half of the squash. Scoop out the flesh to make room for the stuffing. Coat the squash half with 1 teaspoon of olive oil.

2. Put the squash half in the perforated pan.

3. Select Bake. Set temperature to 350ºF (180ºC) and set time to 15 minutes. Press Start to begin preheating.

4. Once preheated, place the pan into the oven. Flip the squash halfway through.

5. When cooking is complete, the squash should be tender.

6. Meanwhile, thoroughly combine the tomatoes, poblano pepper, remaining 1 teaspoon of olive oil, salt, and pepper in a bowl.

7. Remove the pan from the oven and spoon the tomato mixture into the squash. Return to the oven.

8. Select Roast. Set time to 15 minutes. Place the pan into the oven

9. After 12 minutes, remove the pan from the oven. Scatter the Mozzarella cheese on top. Return the pan to the oven and continue cooking.

10. When cooking is complete, the tomatoes should be soft and the cheese should be melted.

11. Cool for 5 minutes before serving.

Nutrition: Calories 79 Carbs 7 g Protein 5 g Fat 3 g

DINNER

Monkfish with Olives and Capers

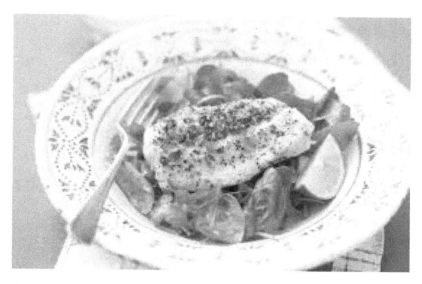

Preparation Time: 20 Minutes

Cooking Time: 45 Minutes

Servings: 4

Ingredients:

- One monkfish
- Ten cherry tomatoes

- 50 g cailletier olives
- Five capers

Directions:

1. Spread aluminum foil inside the basket and place the monkfish clean and skinless.
2. Add chopped tomatoes, olives, capers, oil, and salt.
3. Set the temperature to 1600C.
4. Cook the monkfish for around 40 minutes.

Nutrition: Calories 404 Fat 29g Carbohydrates 36g Sugars 7g Protein 24g Cholesterol 36mg

Shrimp, Zucchini and Cherry Tomato Sauce

Preparation Time: 10 Minutes

Cooking Time: 30 Minutes

Servings: 4

Ingredients:

- Two zucchinis
- 300 shrimp
- Seven cherry tomatoes
- Salt to taste
- One clove garlic

Directions:

1. Pour the oil, add the garlic clove, and diced zucchini.
2. Cook for 15 minutes at 1500C.
3. Add the shrimp and the pieces of tomato, salt, and spices.
4. Cook for another 5 to 10 minutes or until the shrimp water evaporates.

Nutrition: Calories 214.3 Fat 8.6g Carbohydrate 7.8g Sugars 4.8g Protein 27.0g Cholesterol 232.7mg

---

Salmon with Pistachio Bark

Preparation Time: 20 Minutes

Cooking Time: 30 Minutes

Servings: 4

Ingredients:

- 600 g salmon fillet
- 50g pistachios
- Salt to taste

Directions:

1. Place the parchment paper on the bottom of the basket and place the salmon fillet in it (it can be cooked whole or already divided into four portions).
2. Cut the pistachios into thick pieces; grease the top of the fish, salt (little because the pistachios are already salted), and cover everything with the pistachios.
3. Set the air fryer to 1800C and simmer for 25 minutes.

Nutrition: Calories 371.7 Fat 21.8 g Carbohydrate 9.4 g Sugars 2.2g Protein 34.7 g Cholesterol 80.5 mg

Salmon in Papillote With Orange

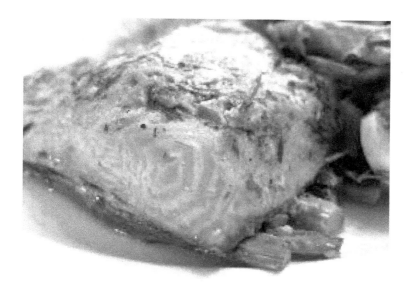

Preparation Time: 20 Minutes

Cooking Time: 30 Minutes

Servings: 4

Ingredients:

- 600g salmon fillet
- Four oranges
- Two cloves of garlic
- Chives to taste
- One lemon

Directions:

1. Pour the freshly squeezed orange juice, the lemon juice, the zest of the two oranges into a bowl. Add two tablespoons of oil, salt, and garlic. Dip the previously washed salmon fillet and leave it in the marinade for one hour, preferably in the refrigerator

2. Place the steak and part of your marinade on a sheet of foil. Salt and sprinkle with chives and a few slices of orange.

3. Set to 1600C. Simmer for 30 minutes. Open the sheet, let it evaporate, and serve with a nice garnish of fresh orange.

Nutrition: Calories 229 Fat 11g Carbohydrates 5g Sugar 3g Protein 25g Cholesterol 62mg

Salted Marinated Salmon

Preparation Time: 10 Minutes

Cooking Time: 30 Minutes

Servings: 2

Ingredients:

- 500g salmon fillet
- 1 kg of coarse salt

Directions:

1. Place the baking paper on the basket and the salmon on top (skin side up) covered with coarse salt.

2. Set the air fryer to 1500C.

3. Cook everything for 25 to 30 minutes. At the end of cooking, remove the salt from the fish and serve with a drizzle of oil.

Nutrition: Calories 290 Fat 13g Carbohydrates 3g Fiber 0g Protein 40g Cholesterol 196mg

Sautéed Trout with Almonds

Preparation Time: 30 Minutes

Cooking Time: 30 Minutes

Servings: 4

Ingredients:

- 700 g salmon trout
- 15 black peppercorns
- Dill leaves to taste
- 30g almonds
- Salt to taste

Directions:

1. Cut the trout into cubes and marinate it for half an hour with the ingredients (except salt).
2. Cook for 17 minutes at 1600C. Pour a drizzle of oil and serve.

Nutrition: Calories 238.5 Fat 20.1 g Carbohydrate 11.5 g Sugars 1.0 g Protein4.0 g Cholesterol 45.9 mg

Stuffed Cuttlefish

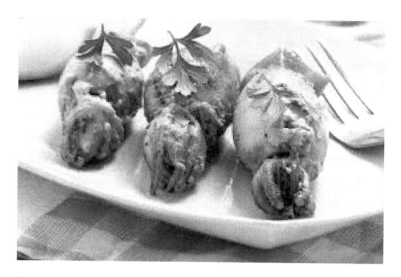

Preparation Time: 20 Minutes

Cooking Time: 30 Minutes

Servings: 4

Ingredients:

- Eight small cuttlefish
- 50 g of breadcrumbs
- Garlic to taste
- Parsley to taste
- One egg

Directions:

1. Clean the cuttlefish, cut, and separate the tentacles. In a blender, pour the breadcrumbs,

the parsley (without the branches), the egg, the salt, a drizzle of olive oil, and the sepia tentacles.

2. Blend until you get a dense mixture. Fill the sepia with the mixture obtained.

3. Place the cuttlefish in the bowl.

4. Set the air fryer to 1500C and cook for 20 minutes. At the end of cooking, add a drizzle of olive oil and serve.

Nutrition: Calories 67.1 Fat 0.6g Carbohydrates 0.7g Protein 13.8g Cholesterol 95.2mg

Rabas

Preparation Time: 5 Minutes

Cooking Time: 12 Minutes

Servings: 4

Ingredients:

- 16 rabas
- One egg
- Breadcrumbs
- Salt, pepper, sweet paprika

Directions:

1. Put the rabas boil for 2 minutes.
2. Remove and dry well.
3. Beat the egg and season to taste. You can put salt, pepper, and sweet paprika—place in the egg.
4. Bread with breadcrumbs. Place in sticks.
5. Place in the fryer for 5 minutes at 1600C. Remove
6. Spray with a cooking spray and place five more minutes at 2000C.

Nutrition: Calories 200 Fat 1g Carbohydrates 1g Sugars 0g Protein 1g Cholesterol 0mg

Garlicky Pork Tenderloin

Preparation Time: 15 Minutes

Cooking Time: 20 Minutes

Servings: 5

Ingredients:

- 1½ pounds pork tenderloin
- Nonstick cooking spray
- Two small heads of roasted garlic
- Salt and ground black pepper, as required

Directions:

1. Lightly spray all the pork sides with cooking spray and then season with salt and black pepper.

2. Now, rub the pork with roasted garlic. Arrange the roast onto the lightly greased cooking tray.

3. Select "Air Fry" and then regulate the temperature to 400 degrees F. Set the timer for 20 minutes and press the "Start."

4. When the display demonstrates "Add Food," insert the cooking tray in the center position.

5. If the display shows "Turn Food," turn the pork.

6. When cooking time is done, remove the tray from Vortex.

7. Place the roast onto a platter for about 10 minutes before slicing.

8. With a sharp knife, cut the roast into desired sized slices and serve.

Nutrition: Calories 202 Fat 4.8 g Carbs 1.7 g Protein 35.9 g

Foil-Packet Lobster Tail

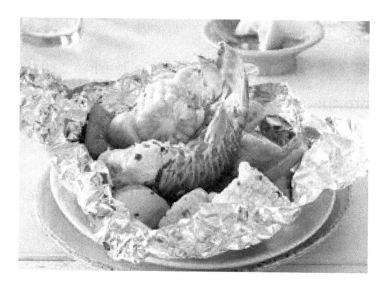

Preparation time: 15 minutes

Cooking time: 12 minutes

Servings: 2

Ingredients:

- 2 (6-ounce) lobster tails, halved
- 2 tablespoons salted butter, melted
- ½ teaspoon old bay seasoning
- Juice of ½ medium lemon
- 1 teaspoon dried parsley

Directions:

1. Place the two halved tails on a sheet of aluminum foil. Drizzle with butter, old bay seasoning, and lemon juice.
2. Seal the foil packets, completely covering tails. Place into the air fryer basket.
3. Adjust the temperature to 375°f and set the timer for 12 minutes.
4. Once done, sprinkle with dried parsley and serve immediately.

Nutrition: Calories: 234 Protein: 28.3 g Fiber: 0.1 g Net carbohydrates: 0.6 g Fat: 11.9 g Sodium: 951 mg Carbohydrates: 0.7 g Sugar: 0.2 g

SNACKS

Prosciutto-Wrapped Guacamole Rings

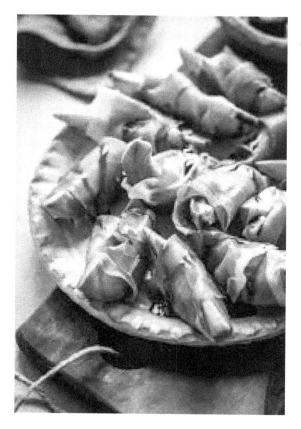

Preparation time: 10 minutes

Cooking time: 6 minutes

Servings: 8 rings

Ingredients:

- 2 avocados, halved, pitted, and peeled
- 3 tablespoons lime juice, plus more to taste
- 2 small plum tomatoes, diced
- ½ cup finely diced onions
- 2 small cloves garlic, smashed to a paste
- 3 tablespoons chopped fresh cilantro leaves
- ½ scant teaspoon fine sea salt
- ½ scant teaspoon ground cumin
- 2 small onions (about 1½-inches in diameter), cut into ½-inch-thick slices
- 8 slices prosciutto

Directions:

1. Make the guacamole: Place the avocados and lime juice in a large bowl and mash with a fork until it reaches your desired consistency. Add the tomatoes, onions, garlic, cilantro, salt, and cumin and stir until well combined. Taste and add more lime juice if desired. Set aside half of the guacamole for serving. (Note: If you're

making the guacamole ahead of time, place it in a large resealable plastic bag, squeeze out all the air, and seal it shut. It will keep in the refrigerator for up to 3 days when stored this way.)

2. Place a piece of parchment paper on a tray that fits in your freezer and place the onion slices on it, breaking the slices apart into 8 rings. Fill each ring with about 2 tablespoons of guacamole. Place the tray in the freezer for 2 hours.

3. Spray the air fryer basket with avocado oil. Preheat the air fryer to 400°F (205°C).

4. Remove the rings from the freezer and wrap each in a slice of prosciutto. Place them in the air fryer basket, leaving space between them (if you're using a smaller air fryer, work in batches if necessary), and cook for 6 minutes, flipping halfway through. Use a spatula to remove the rings from the air fryer. Serve with the reserved half of the guacamole.

5. Store leftovers in an airtight container in the refrigerator for up to 4 days. Reheat in a

preheated 400°F (205ºC) air fryer for about 3 minutes, until heated through.

Nutrition: calories: 132 fat: 9g protein: 5g carbs: 10g net carbs: 6g fiber: 4g

Cheesy Pork Rind Tortillas

Preparation time: 10 minutes

Cooking time: 5 minutes

Servings: 4 tortillas

Ingredients:

- 1 ounce (28 g) pork rinds
- ¾ cup shredded Mozzarella cheese
- 2 tablespoons full-fat cream cheese
- 1 large egg

Directions:

1. Place pork rinds into food processor and pulse until finely ground.

2. Place Mozzarella into a large microwave-safe bowl. Break cream cheese into small pieces and add them to the bowl. Microwave for 30 seconds, or until both cheeses are melted and can easily be stirred together into a ball. Add ground pork rinds and egg to the cheese mixture.

3. Continue stirring until the mixture forms a ball. If it cools too much and cheese hardens, microwave for 10 more seconds.

4. Separate the dough into four small balls. Place each ball of dough between two sheets of parchment and roll into ¼-inch flat layer.

5. Place tortillas into the air fryer basket in single layer, working in batches if necessary.

6. Adjust the temperature to 400°F (205ºC) and set the timer for 5 minutes.

7. Tortillas will be crispy and firm when fully cooked. Serve immediately.

Nutrition: calories: 145 fat: 10g protein: 11g carbs: 1g net carbs: 1g fiber: 0g

Cheesy Pork and Chicken

Preparation time: 5 minutes

Cooking time: 5 minutes

Servings: 2

Ingredients:

- 1 ounce (28 g) pork rinds
- 4 ounces (113 g) shredded cooked chicken
- ½ cup shredded Monterey jack cheese
- ¼ cup sliced pickled jalapeños
- ¼ cup guacamole
- ¼ cup full-fat sour cream

Directions:

1. Place pork rinds into 6-inch round baking pan. Cover with shredded chicken and Monterey jack cheese. Place pan into the air fryer basket.

2. Adjust the temperature to 370°F (188°C) and set the timer for 5 minutes or until cheese is melted.

3. Top with jalapeños, guacamole, and sour cream. Serve immediately.

Nutrition: calories: 395 fat: 27g protein: 30g carbs: 3g net carbs: 2g fiber: 1g

Pork Cheese Sticks

Preparation time: 20 minutes

Cooking time: 10 minutes

Servings: 12 sticks

Ingredients:

- 6 (1-ounce / 28-g) Mozzarella string cheese sticks
- ½ cup grated Parmesan cheese
- ½ ounce (14 g) pork rinds, finely ground
- 1 teaspoon dried parsley
- 2 large eggs

Directions:

1. Place Mozzarella sticks on a cutting board and cut in half. Freeze 45 minutes or until firm. If freezing overnight, remove frozen sticks after 1 hour and place into airtight zip-top storage bag and place back in freezer for future use.
2. In a large bowl, mix Parmesan, ground pork rinds, and parsley.
3. In a medium bowl, whisk eggs.

4. Dip a frozen Mozzarella stick into beaten eggs and then into Parmesan mixture to coat. Repeat with remaining sticks. Place Mozzarella sticks into the air fryer basket.

5. Adjust the temperature to 400°F (205ºC) and set the timer for 10 minutes or until golden.

6. Serve warm.

Nutrition: calories: 236 fat: 13g protein: 19g carbs: 5g net carbs: 5gfiber: 0g

Cheesy Cauliflower Buns

Preparation time: 15 minutes

Cooking time: 12 minutes

Servings: 8 buns

Ingredients:

- 1 (12-ounce 340-g) steamer bag cauliflower, cooked according to package instructions
- ½ cup shredded Mozzarella cheese
- ¼ cup shredded mild Cheddar cheese
- ¼ cup blanched finely ground almond flour
- 1 large egg
- ½ teaspoon salt

Directions:

1. Let cooked cauliflower cool about 10 minutes. Use a kitchen towel to wring out excess moisture, then place cauliflower in a food processor.
2. Add Mozzarella, Cheddar, flour, egg, and salt to the food processor and pulse twenty times until mixture is combined. It will resemble a soft, wet dough.

3. Divide mixture into eight piles. Wet your hands with water to prevent sticking, then press each pile into a flat bun shape, about ½-inch thick.

4. Cut a sheet of parchment to fit air fryer basket. Working in batches if needed, place the formed dough onto ungreased parchment in air fryer basket. Adjust the temperature to 350°F (180ºC) and set the timer for 12 minutes, turning buns halfway through cooking.

5. Let buns cool 10 minutes before serving. Serve warm.

Nutrition: calories: 75 fat: 5g protein: 5g carbs: 3g net carbs: 2g fiber: 1g

Bacon Cauliflower Skewers

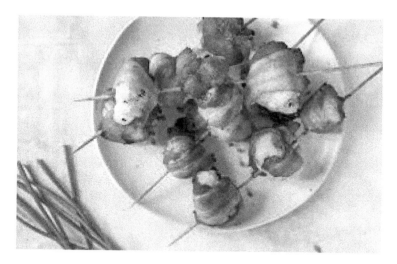

Preparation time: 10 minutes

Cooking time: 12 minutes

Servings: 4

Ingredients:

- 4 slices sugar-free bacon, cut into thirds
- ¼ medium yellow onion, peeled and cut into 1-inch pieces
- 4 ounces (113 g) (about 8) cauliflower florets
- 1½ tablespoons olive oil
- ¼ teaspoon salt
- ¼ teaspoon garlic powder

Directions:

1. Place 1 piece bacon and 2 pieces onion on a 6-inch skewer. Add a second piece bacon, and 2 cauliflower florets, followed by another piece of bacon onto skewer. Repeat with remaining ingredients and three additional skewers to make four total skewers.
2. Drizzle skewers with olive oil, then sprinkle with salt and garlic powder. Place skewers into ungreased air fryer basket. Adjust the temperature to 375°F (190ºC) and set the timer for 12 minutes, turning the skewers halfway through cooking. When done, vegetables will be tender and bacon will be crispy. Serve warm.

Nutrition: calories: 69 fat: 5g protein: 5g carbs: 2g net carbs: 1g fiber: 1g

Crispy Cheese Salami Roll-Ups

Preparation time: 5 minutes

Cooking time: 4 minutes

Servings: 16 roll-ups

Ingredients:

- 4 ounces (113 g) cream cheese, broken into 16 equal pieces
- 16 (0.5-ounce / 14-g) deli slices Genoa salami

Directions:

1. Place a piece of cream cheese at the edge of a slice of salami and roll to close. Secure with a toothpick. Repeat with remaining cream cheese pieces and salami.
2. Place roll-ups in an ungreased 6-inch round nonstick baking dish and place into air fryer basket. Adjust the temperature to 350°F (180ºC) and set the timer for 4 minutes. Salami will be crispy and cream cheese will be warm when done. Let cool 5 minutes before serving.

Nutrition: calories: 269 fat: 22g protein: 11g carbs: 2g net carbs: 2g fiber: 0g

Cheesy Zucchini Fries

Preparation time: 10 minutes

Cooking time: 10 minutes

Servings: 8

Ingredients:

- 2 medium zucchinis, ends removed, quartered lengthwise, and sliced into 3-inch-long fries
- ½ teaspoon salt
- $^1/_3$ cup heavy whipping cream
- ½ cup blanched finely ground almond flour
- ¾ cup grated Parmesan cheese
- 1 teaspoon Italian seasoning

Directions:

1. Sprinkle zucchini with salt and wrap in a kitchen towel to draw out excess moisture. Let sit 2 hours.
2. Pour cream into a medium bowl. In a separate medium bowl, whisk together flour, Parmesan, and Italian seasoning.
3. Place each zucchini fry into cream, then gently shake off excess. Press each fry into dry

mixture, coating each side, then place into ungreased air fryer basket. Adjust the temperature to 400°F (205ºC) and set the timer for 10 minutes, turning fries halfway through cooking. Fries will be golden and crispy when done. Place on clean parchment sheet to cool 5 minutes before serving.

Nutrition: calories: 124 fat: 10g protein: 5g carbs: 4g net carbs: 3g fiber: 1g

Aromatic Avocado Fries

Preparation time: 10 minutes

Cooking time: 15 minutes

Servings: 6

Ingredients:

- 3 firm, barely ripe avocados, halved, peeled, and pitted
- 2 cups pork dust (or powdered Parmesan cheese for vegetarian;)
- 2 teaspoons fine sea salt
- 2 teaspoons ground black pepper
- 2 teaspoons ground cumin
- 1 teaspoon chili powder
- 1 teaspoon paprika
- ½ teaspoon garlic powder
- ½ teaspoon onion powder
- 2 large eggs
- Salsa, for serving (optional)
- Fresh chopped cilantro leaves, for garnish (optional)

Directions:

1. Spray the air fryer basket with avocado oil. Preheat the air fryer to 400°F (205°C).

2. Slice the avocados into thick-cut French fry shapes.

3. In a bowl, mix together the pork dust, salt, pepper, and seasonings.

4. In a separate shallow bowl, beat the eggs.

5. Dip the avocado fries into the beaten eggs and shake off any excess, then dip them into the pork dust mixture. Use your hands to press the breading into each fry.

6. Spray the fries with avocado oil and place them in the air fryer basket in a single layer, leaving space between them. If there are too many fries to fit in a single layer, work in batches. Cook in the air fryer for 13 to 15 minutes, until golden brown, flipping after 5 minutes.

7. Serve with salsa, if desired, and garnish with fresh chopped cilantro, if desired. Best served fresh.

8. Store leftovers in an airtight container in the fridge for up to 5 days. Reheat in a preheated

400°F (205ºC) air fryer for 3 minutes, or until heated through.

Nutrition: calories: 282 fat: 22g protein: 15g carbs: 9g net carbs: 2g fiber: 7g

Cheesy Pickle Spear

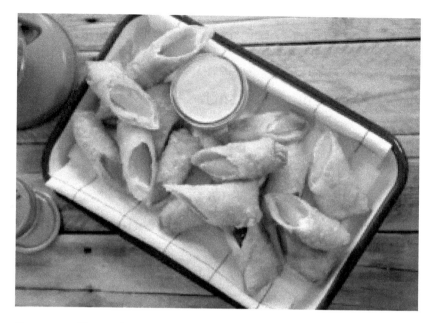

Preparation time: 40 minutes

Cooking time: 10 minutes

Servings: 4

Ingredients:

- 4 dill pickle spears, halved lengthwise
- ¼ cup ranch dressing
- ½ cup blanched finely ground almond flour
- ½ cup grated Parmesan cheese
- 2 tablespoons dry ranch seasoning

Directions:

1. Wrap spears in a kitchen towel 30 minutes to soak up excess pickle juice.

2. Pour ranch dressing into a medium bowl and add pickle spears. In a separate medium bowl, mix flour, Parmesan, and ranch seasoning.

3. Remove each spear from ranch dressing and shake off excess. Press gently into dry mixture to coat all sides. Place spears into ungreased air fryer basket. Adjust the temperature to 400°F (205ºC) and set the timer for 10 minutes, turning spears three times during cooking. Serve warm.

Nutrition: calories: 160 fat: 11g protein: 7gcarbs: 8g net carbs: 6g fiber: 2g

DESSERTS

Raspberry Bars

Preparation Time: 10 Minutes

Cooking Time: 6 Minutes

Servings: 12

Ingredients:

- ½ cup coconut butter, melted
- ½ cup of coconut oil
- ½ cup raspberries, dried
- ¼ cup swerve
- ½ cup coconut, shredded

Directions:

1. In your food processor, blend dried berries very well.
2. In a bowl that fits your air fryer, mix oil with butter, swerve, coconut and raspberries, toss

well, introduce in the fryer and cook at 320 degrees F for 6 minutes.

3. Spread this on a lined baking sheet, keep in the fridge for an hour, slice, and serve.

4. Enjoy!

Nutrition: Calories 164 Fat 22 Fiber 2 Carbs 4 Protein 2

Cocoa Berries Cream

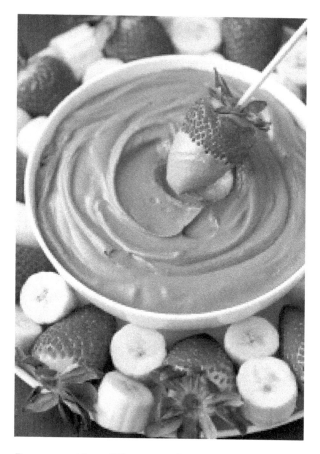

Preparation Time: 10 Minutes

Cooking Time: 10 Minutes

Servings: 4

Ingredients:

- Three tablespoons cocoa powder
- 14 ounces coconut cream

- 1 cup blackberries
- 1 cup raspberries
- Two tablespoons stevia

Directions:

1. In a bowl, whisk cocoa powder with stevia and cream and stir.
2. Add raspberries and blackberries, toss gently, transfer to a pan that fits your air fryer, introduce in the fryer, and cook at 350 degrees F for 10 minutes.
3. Divide into bowls and serve cold.
4. Enjoy!

Nutrition: Calories 205 Fat 34 Fiber 2 Carbs 6 Protein 2

Cocoa Pudding

Preparation Time: 10 Minutes

Cooking Time: 20 Minutes

Servings: 2

Ingredients:

- Two tablespoons water
- ½ tablespoon agar
- Four tablespoons stevia
- Four tablespoons cocoa powder
- 2 cups coconut milk, hot

Directions:

1. In a bowl, mix milk with stevia and cocoa powder and stir well.
2. In a bowl, mix agar with water, stir well, add to the cocoa mix, stir and transfer to a pudding pan that fits your air fryer.
3. Introduce in the fryer and cook at 356 degrees F for 20 minutes.
4. Serve the pudding cold.
5. Enjoy!

Nutrition: Calories 170 Fat 2 Fiber 1 Carbs 4 Protein 3

Blueberry Coconut Crackers

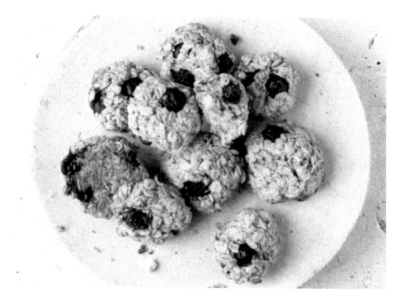

Preparation Time: 10 Minutes

Cooking Time: 30 Minutes

Servings: 12

Ingredients:

- ½ cup coconut butter
- ½ cup coconut oil, melted
- 1 cup blueberries
- Three tablespoons coconut sugar

Directions:

1. Mix coconut butter with coconut oil, raspberries, and sugar, toss, introduce in the fryer and cook at 367 degrees F for 30 minutes
2. Spread on a lined baking sheet, keep in the fridge for a few hours, slice crackers, and serve.
3. Enjoy!

Nutrition: Calories 174 Fat 5 Fiber 2 Carbs 4 Protein 7

Cauliflower Pudding

Preparation Time: 10 Minutes

Cooking Time: 30 Minutes

Servings: 4

Ingredients:

- Two and ½ cups of water
- 1 cup of coconut sugar
- 2 cups cauliflower rice
- Two cinnamon sticks
- ½ cup coconut, shredded

Directions:

1. Mix water with coconut sugar, cauliflower rice, cinnamon, and coconut, stir, introduce in the fryer, then cook using 365 degrees F for 30 minutes
2. Divide pudding into cups and serve cold.
3. Enjoy!

Nutrition: Calories 203 Fat 4 Fiber 6 Carbs 9 Protein 4

Sweet Vanilla Rhubarb

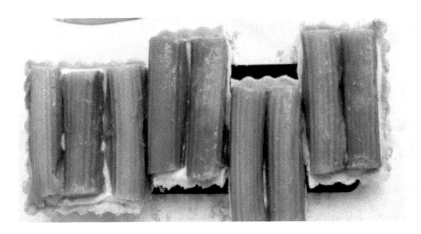

Preparation Time: 10 Minutes

Cooking Time: 10 Minutes

Servings: 4

Ingredients:

- 5 cups rhubarb, chopped
- Two tablespoons coconut butter, melted
- 1/3 cup water
- One tablespoon stevia
- One teaspoon vanilla extract

Directions:

1. Put rhubarb, ghee, water, stevia, and vanilla extract in a pan that fits your air fryer, set up in

the fryer, and cook at 365 degrees F for 10 minutes

2. Divide into small bowls and serve cold.

3. Enjoy!

Nutrition: Calories 103 Fat 2 Fiber 1 Carbs 6 Protein 2

Pineapple and Apricots

Preparation Time: 10 Minutes

Cooking Time: 12 Minutes

Servings: 10

Ingredients:

- 6 cups canned pineapple chunks, drained
- 4 cups canned apricots, halved and drained
- 3 cups natural applesauce
- 2 cups canned mandarin oranges, drained
- Two tablespoons stevia

Directions:

1. Put pineapples, apricots, applesauce, oranges, cinnamon, and stevia in a pan that fits your air fryer, introduce in the fryer, and cook at 360 degrees F for 12 minutes.
2. Divide into small bowls and serve cold.
3. Enjoy!

Nutrition: Calories 130 Fat 1 Fiber 2 Carbs 7 Protein 2

Low Carb Peanut Butter Cookies

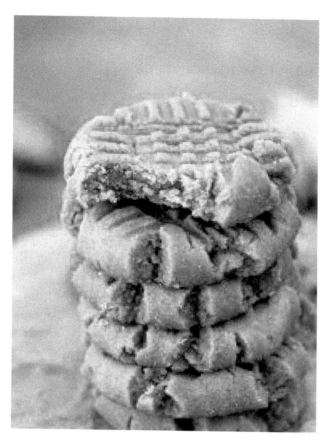

Preparation Time: 5 Minutes

Cooking Time: 25 Minutes

Servings: 27

Ingredients:

- Two large eggs
- ½ cup erythritol
- One ¼ cup creamy peanut butter

- ¾ cup peanuts
- ¼ tsp. Salt

Directions:

1. Crush the peanuts and set aside. Preheat the oven to 350 degrees and use a cookie sheet covered with parchment paper.

2. Combine eggs, sweetener, salt, and creamy peanut butter in a blender or food processor. Manage until smooth and clean offsides when mixture sticks.

3. Toss in crushed peanuts and join with other ingredients. Leave some crunch for texture.

4. Scoop the dough into spheres and place them on a baking sheet.

5. Press the dough using a fork to create a crosshatch top. Wipe fork with water before using it again.

6. Bake for 20 minutes or wait until golden brown and crunchy.

Nutrition: Calories: 94 Protein: 4g Net Carbs: 2g Fat 7g

Strawberry Cheesecake Chimichangas

Preparation Time: 15 Minutes

Cooking Time: 10 Minutes

Servings: 6

Ingredients:

- 6 (8-inch) soft flour tortillas
- 8 ounces cream cheese
- Two tablespoons sour cream
- One teaspoon vanilla extract
- 3/4 cups strawberries

Directions:

1. Allow the cream cheese to soften and slice your strawberries into thin slices.
2. Beat together cream cheese, vanilla, sugar, and sour cream.
3. Fold the strawberries into the mixture.
4. Spread the filling on the bottom 1/3 of each tortilla.
5. Fold the bottom and top of the tortilla in, then roll it up from the sides.

6. Cook at 340 for about 8 minutes or until the tortillas become crisp.

7. Allow cooling a few minutes before serving.

Nutrition: Calories: 296 Sodium: 574 mg Dietary Fiber: 5.4g Fat: 18.1g Carbs: 27.7g Protein: 8.1g

Monkey Bread

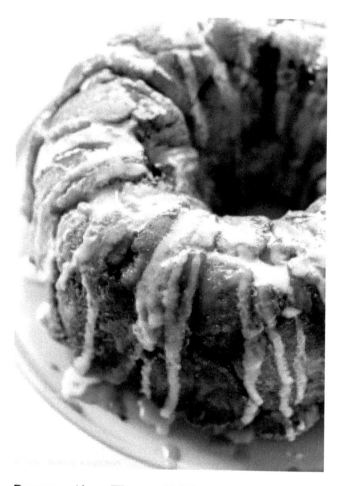

Preparation Time: 7 Minutes

Cooking Time: 7 Minutes

Servings: 4

Ingredients:

- 1 cup self-rising flour

- 1 cup non-fat Greek yogurt

- One teaspoon sugar

- 1/2 teaspoon cinnamon

Directions:

1. Mix the flour and yogurt until it forms a dough.

2. Roll the dough and form a circle, then cut it into fourths.

3. Flatten each quarter and cut it into eight pieces.

4. Roll the pieces into balls.

5. Combine cinnamon and sugar into a bag and shake well to mix.

6. Add eight balls to the bag and shake to cover.

7. Preheat the fryer to 375 degrees.

8. Put the balls in a loaf pan that fits your basket.

9. Cook in your fryer for 7 minutes.

Nutrition: Calories:151 Sodium: 46 mg Dietary Fiber: 1.7g Fat: .0.3g Carbs: 30.3g Protein: 6.2g

CONCLUSION

Thanks, once again for reaching the end of this book Air Fryer Cookbook.

Air Fryer is a kitchen device that is introduced by the famous TV chef, Emeril Lagasse. It can cook and fry any variety of chicken, turkey, fish, meat, vegetables or even bake bread, cake or pie. It can cook the same dish with different flavors. To give the same dish different flavors, it only needs to be placed in the food chamber more than one time. It saves time and does not make any mess to clean up. The recipe book Air Fryer Cookbook includes the best recipes that can be cooked using this new machine.

Air frying technology had existed for quite time but it was introduced by this new breakthrough technology. It was introduced in 2012 as food cooking product. Emeril Lagasse was the first to demonstrate the use of this technology in the field of food, the food industry level. It improved the quality of food produced in different kitchens with minimum energy usage. Large bowls and food cookers were replaced with new air fryer, which was able to produce as much fish as was cooked in 20 minutes. Its energy consumption is high but it saves a lot of time. This device is very useful for fast food users. It cooks food faster without causing the food to go bad.

Now, that you had encountered the recipes in this book, I hope you've enjoyed the time you had spent with us and hope you begin using our recipes to cook in your air fryers.

We are not done yet; I'd like you to perform some simple more common habits when using your Air Fryer to make cooking easier and more efficient:

1. Cut vegetables into appropriate sizes before you start cooking them.
2. Wash and peel vegetables prior to cutting.
3. To soften vegetables, use steam, boiled water or baking soda and not for too long.
4. Be Healthy by adding as little oil as possible in each recipe.
5. Do not deep fry for more than 10 minutes.
6. To check if your food is cooked, it should flex easily.
7. If you are using aluminum foil to contain the oil, do not forget to re-iron it every time you air fry.
8. To remove the odor from your hands, wash them with vinegar or lemon juice before you start cooking.
9. To remove the remaining smell of smoked food (e.g., fish) Fry some onions to remove the smell.

Here are some more habits that you should avoid:

1. Do not heat oils.
2. Do not reheat food.

3. Do not use too much oil; just the perfect amount.

4. Do not overcook foods.

5. Do not use boiling water; it could get stuck in your fryer.

6. Do not overfill your fryer.

7. Do not stack meats or vegetables.

8. Do not keep the greasy food for long time.

9. Do not keep your food in the utensils that have been used for stews or stinking foods.

10. Do not use aluminum foil, if you are not cooking with oil.

Thank you again for purchasing this book and goodbye for now.

Best of Luck on your choice and enjoy the air fryer cooking.

CPSIA information can be obtained
at www.ICGtesting.com
Printed in the USA
BVHW051758120421
604747BV00011B/739